Nursing & Health Survival Guide

Recognising the Acutely Ill Child

Elizabeth Charnock
Angela Lee
Amanda Miller

T0033793

First published 2013 by Pearson Education Limited

Published 2014 by Routledge
2 Park Square, Milton Park, Abingdon, Oxon OX14 4RN
711 Third Avenue, New York, NY 10017, USA

Routledge is an imprint of the Taylor & Francis Group, an informa business

ISBN 13: 978-0-273-76372-7 (hbk)

British Library Cataloguing-in-Publication Data
A catalogue record for this book is available from the British Library

Library of Congress Cataloging-in-Publication Data
Charnock, Elizabeth, 1969-
    Recognising the acutely ill child / Elizabeth Charnock, Angela Lee, Amanda Miller.
       p. ; cm. -- (Nursing & health survival guide)
    Includes bibliographical references.
    ISBN 978-0-273-76372-7
    I. Lee, Angela, 1966- II. Miller, Amanda, 1975- III. Title. IV. Series: Nursing
& health survival guides.
       [DNLM: 1. Pediatric Nursing--methods--Handbooks. 2. Child. 3. Critical
Care--methods--Handbooks. WY49]
    LC Classification not assigned
    618.92'00231--dc23
                                                                        2012016935

Typeset in 8/9.5pt Helvetica by 35

Printed in the UK by Severn, Gloucester on responsibly sourced paper

MIX
Paper | Supporting
responsible forestry
FSC® C022174

contents

INTRODUCTION: THE IMPORTANCE OF EARLY RECOGNITION OF ACUTE ILLNESS IN CHILDREN	1
KEY PRINCIPLES OF PHYSICAL ASSESSMENT	2
Standards for assessing and measuring physiological observations	2
Temperature	4
Pulse and respiration	4
Blood pressure	5
Recording physiological observations	6
The limitations of Early Warning Scores (EWS)	6
The importance of parental observations	7
CHILDREN ARE DIFFERENT FROM ADULTS	8
Pre-terminal signs	8
Anatomical and physiological differences between children and adults	8
A structured approach to assessment	11
ASSESSMENT OF AIRWAY (A)	12
Is the airway open?	12
Are there any added sounds which may indicate airway difficulties?	13
Airway adjuncts	13
ASSESSMENT OF BREATHING (B)	14
Effort of breathing	15
Efficacy of breathing	18
Effects of breathing inadequacy on other organs	20
Respiratory severity assessment	20
Oxygen delivery adjuncts	21
ASSESSMENT OF CIRCULATION (C)	23
Heart rate	23
Pulse volume	24
Pulse rhythm	24
Capillary refill time (CRT) and body temperature	25
Blood pressure	26
Recognising the shocked child	26
Classification and causes of shock	27
The three stages of shock	28
Meningococcal septicaemia: signs and symptoms	30
Recognising the dehydrated child	31
Calculation of fluid requirements	33
ASSESSMENT OF DISABILITY (D)	34
Rapid assessment of disability: AVPU	34
Posture	36
Pupils	37

Causes of raised intracranial pressure
Signs of raised intracranial pressure
Seizures
'Don't ever forget glucose': DEFG
Tips to promote accurate measurement and recording of neurological
observations
Contraindications to performing a lumbar puncture
ASSESSMENT OF EXPOSURE (E)
Rashes and bruising
Temperature
APPENDICES
1 Physiological observations: normal ranges and estimation of
weight formula
2 Paediatric SBAR tool
3 Basic life support – paediatric algorithm
4 Paediatric FBAO treatment algorithm
REFERENCES
USEFUL WEBSITES

The importance of early recognition of acute illness in children

An analysis of patient deaths (NPSA 2007) highlighted the failure of nursing and medical staff to recognise early deterioration in patients as contributing to delays in summoning and initiating effective intervention with appropriate urgency. With specific reference to the care of children, the report *Why Children Die* (CEMACH 2008, Key Finding 3) identified delay and problems in recognising serious illness in children as a concern. The message is clear: **early recognition of acute illness in children may help to improve patient outcomes and may save lives.**

Accurate and prompt assessment is required in order to:

- provide an accurate baseline for comparison of future observations
- contribute to the accurate diagnosis of the child's condition
- ensure early recognition of the acutely ill child
- promptly spot deterioration of the child's condition
- trigger early review and effective management of the child's condition.

Key principles of physical assessment

■ STANDARDS FOR ASSESSING AND MEASURING PHYSIOLOGICAL OBSERVATIONS

Prompt recognition of the acutely ill child relies on the skilful and competent assessment and measurement of physiological observations performed with accuracy and attention to detail.

- Assessment of the child should start before any direct contact is made. Prior to approaching the child, observe them from afar, noting their uninterrupted behaviour, play and movements, and their interaction with parents. Record and report any concerns.
- Use the four senses of sight, hearing/listening, touch and smell (Table 1) to elicit important information about the child's health (Glasper, McEwing and Richardson 2011).
- Physiological observations may be a source of anxiety and concern for both the child and parents. Compassionate and respectful care demands that observations are preceded by gaining consent and are accompanied by an explanation of both the procedure and its results.
- Physiological monitoring equipment should be used as instructed by the manufacturers, paying specific attention to the correct sizing, positioning and use of probes, cuffs and leads. **Remember: inappropriate and incorrect use of equipment is likely to yield inaccurate observations which may contribute to the late or non-recognition of acute illness in the child.**
- You are responsible and accountable for the quality and reliability of physiological observations performed by you.

You must ensure that physiological observations are interpreted accurately, if not by you then by someone else. **Follow local policies and guidelines, and seek help when unsure.**

Table 1

Sight	Initial eyeballing – does the child look sick? Are there any obvious injuries? How are they behaving? Are they interacting with parents? Did they walk into the assessment area? Are they playing? Are they giving eye contact? Are they lethargic? Is the child distressed?
Hearing/ listening	Is the infant crying? A parent may distinguish between a cry of hunger, pain, illness or boredom Are there any respiratory noises present? Is the child talking in sentences?
Touch	Is their skin cold and clammy? Is their skin dry to touch or is there reduced skin turgor? Is the child/infant affectionate with parents?
Smell	Does the child's breath smell? Pear drop smell can indicate diabetic ketoacidosis Is there a smell of alcohol? Does the urine or faeces smell abnormal? Rotavirus has a specific smell Do any wounds have an odour?

■ TEMPERATURE

- All children who present with an acute illness or appear warm to touch or cold and mottled should have their temperature recorded.
- A thermometer appropriate to the age of the infant or child should be used:
  - Less than 4 weeks old, use an electronic thermometer in the axilla (NICE 2007a).
  - From 4 weeks old, use an electronic/chemical dot thermometer in the axilla or a tympanic thermometer (RCN 2011).
  - Oral and rectal thermometers should not be routinely used in children under 5 years of age. Rectal thermometers should only be used under specific guidance dictated and justified by the severity of the child's illness (NICE 2007a).

■ PULSE AND RESPIRATION

- Rather than palpation of a pulse point, use a stethoscope to auscultate the apex heart rate of children less than 2 years of age.
- Heart/pulse and respiration rates should be counted for one full minute to recognise and take into account any normal variations and help detect any abnormalities.
- Electronic data, gained using cardiac or pulse oximeter monitors, should be verified manually by auscultation of the heart rate or palpation of the pulse rate. **Remember: careful interpretation is required to judge the accuracy of electronic data.**

- A full respiratory assessment considering respiratory effort, efficacy and effects on other organs should accompany the measurement of respiratory rate.
- **Remember: not all breath sounds are audible without auscultation. There is a chance that important indicators of respiratory distress will be missed if you do not use a stethoscope to listen for extra breath sounds** (RCN 2011).

BLOOD PRESSURE

- Ideally the child's arm should be used to measure blood pressure (the lower leg may be used in infants when this is not possible).
- It is vital that the blood pressure cuff is correctly sized and positioned:
  - The limb should be well supported at the level of the heart.
  - The cuff width should be more than 80 per cent of the length of the upper arm and the bladder of the cuff should be more than 40 per cent of the arm's circumference (Advanced Life Support Group 2011).
  - The centre of the bladder, from which the leads extend, should cover the brachial artery (Dougherty and Lister 2008).
- Disregard the first reading on an automated blood pressure monitor, as this serves only to regulate the monitor (RCN 2011).
- If blood pressure is consistently recorded as high using an automated blood pressure monitor, confirm the measurement by remeasuring blood pressure manually using a sphygmomanometer (RCN 2011).

■ RECORDING PHYSIOLOGICAL OBSERVATIONS

- The frequency of recording should be directed by local and national policy and the child's individual condition.
- Activity such as sucking, eating/feeding, movement and crying can influence heart rates, respiratory rates and blood pressure, and should therefore be noted alongside physiological observations to ensure accurate interpretation of measurements.
- To aid the accuracy of physiological measurements, document the anatomical sites used to record data and specify the equipment type and size used.
- **Remember: physiological measurements require individualised interpretation; try to find out why the child is presenting with the physiological signs and symptoms recorded. If in any doubt, get immediate help and advice from a senior member of staff.**
- Communicate clearly and assertively all your concerns to ensure that the acutely ill child is treated effectively without delay. The SBAR tool provides a framework to facilitate effective communication (see Appendix 2).

■ THE LIMITATIONS OF EARLY WARNING SCORES (EWS)

Early Warning Scores (EWS) play an important part in aiding the early detection of the acutely ill child, **if review and intervention when triggered is communicated effectively to others and performed without delay. Remember: to be effective, the EWS demands accurate interpretation to overcome its limitations.**

- The EWS needs to be individualised. Question and interpret the observations made in conjunction with a detailed individualised patient history. The EWS may need adapting by an authorised member of the healthcare team to accommodate the child's normal physiological status if outside the parameters of the EWS.
- **Remember: things may not be as they first appear.** For example, respiratory distress may manifest in a low rather than a high respiration rate in the exhausted child prior to collapse. Interrogate the EWS with the child's recent medical history in mind to confirm that it accurately represents the status of the child.
- Check observation trends to spot rapid, rather than gradual falling rates, which may indicate imminent collapse rather than improvement.

THE IMPORTANCE OF PARENTAL OBSERVATIONS

- Involve parents in interpreting the observations made, as they may be able to spot the more subtle and unique signs of deterioration not covered by the EWS.
- Take the concerns and worries of parents seriously; nagging concerns expressed by parents, however vague, should urge you to **stop**, **question** and **review** the child's condition.
- Conveying empathy and compassion to the child and parents will aid the development of a trusting professional relationship. This may help encourage parents and children to voice their opinions, concerns and fears – information that may well be vital to the assessment.

Children are different from adults

■ PRE-TERMINAL SIGNS

Children respond differently to illness than adults, often deteriorating more rapidly. **Remember: if any of the following signs are observed, call for emergency help as the child is in a state of imminent collapse**.

- **Exhaustion:** not to be mistaken for signs of improvement. Rapid reduction in respiratory or heart rates is not necessarily a mark of improvement and may instead indicate exhaustion and pending collapse. Analyse observation trends to ensure accurate interpretation of the child's condition.
- **Bradycardia:** a pulse rate less than 60 beats per minute.
- A rapidly falling heart rate.
- **Gasping:** indicative of severe hypoxia, which leads to bradycardia.
- **Cyanosis:** a late sign of hypoxia.
- **Hypotension:** a late sign of circulatory failure.
- **Absent peripheral and weak central pulses:** a sign of advanced shock.

(Advanced Life Support Group 2011)

■ ANATOMICAL AND PHYSIOLOGICAL DIFFERENCES BETWEEN CHILDREN AND ADULTS

Anatomical and physiological differences between children and adults are detailed in Table 2.

Table 2

ANATOMICAL/PHYSIOLOGICAL FEATURE	POTENTIAL CONSEQUENCES
Large occiput in infants → neck flexion	Airway obstruction
Infant's tongue is larger in proportion to size of mouth	Airway obstruction
Epiglottis is floppy in younger children	Airway closure when conscious level decreased
Trachea in infants short, narrow and soft	More compressible → airway obstruction Increased resistance within airway → respiratory distress
Cricoid ring narrowest point of upper airway compared to vocal cords in adults	If intubation required, risk of oedema, potential sub-glottic stenosis
Smaller upper and lower airways	More easily obstructed by foreign body, mucosal swelling or secretions → Increase in respiratory effort
Reduced number of alveoli until approximately 8 years old	Reduced surface area for gas exchange

⇒

ANATOMICAL/PHYSIOLOGICAL FEATURE	POTENTIAL CONSEQUENCES
Cartilaginous rib cage with ribs lying horizontal that are much more compliant than adults	More compressible → chest recession and reduced efficiency in breathing → infants increase their respiratory rate
Lower percentage of fatigue-resistant type 1 muscle fibres in diaphragm – 25 per cent compared to 50 per cent in adults	Increased susceptibility to fatigue when effort of breathing increases
Diaphragm position is more horizontal than that of adults	Decreased efficiency in contractions
Higher resting metabolic rate	Increased oxygen demand
Immature immune systems	More susceptible to infections
Children preferentially ventilate their upper lobe regions rather than the dependent sections as in adults	In children with unilateral lung disease, placing the non-affected lung uppermost can optimise oxygenation

References / Advanced Life Support Group (2011); Glasper, McEwing and Richardson (2007).

A STRUCTURED APPROACH TO ASSESSMENT

The assessment of a sick child should be carried out using the commonly recognised ABCDE approach. Ask the questions listed in Table 3.

Table 3

Airway	Breathing
<ul><li>Is the airway open?</li><li>Is the infant/child crying/talking?</li><li>Are there any upper airway noises (stridor) indicating upper airway obstruction?</li><li>**Look** – is the chest/abdomen rising and falling?</li><li>**Listen** – are there audible breath sounds?</li><li>**Feel** – can you feel the infant/child's breath on your cheek?</li></ul>	<ul><li>Is the respiratory rate within normal limits?</li><li>Are there signs of recession?</li><li>Are accessory muscles being used?</li><li>Are their inspiratory or expiratory noises present?</li><li>Is grunting or gasping heard?</li><li>Is there nasal flaring?</li><li>Are oxygen saturations within normal limits?</li><li>On auscultation, are breath sounds equal and symmetrical?</li></ul>

⇒

Circulation	Disability

• Is the heart rate within normal limits?
• Are peripheral pulses palpable?
• Is the central pulse weak or bounding?
• Is the capillary refill time < 2 seconds?
• Is blood pressure within normal limits?
	• Is the child/infant:
	  A Alert?
	  V Responsive to Voice?
	  P Responsive to Pain?
	  U Unresponsive?
	• What is the child/infant's blood sugar?
	• Are pupils equal and reactive to light?
	• Is the child/infant's posture normal?

	Exposure
	• Does the child/infant have a fever? • Are there any signs of rashes/bruising?

Assessment of Airway (A)

The patency of the airway is assessed using the **look, listen and feel** approach (Advanced Life Support Group 2011). See Appendix 3 for the Resuscitation Council UK (2010) basic life support algorithm.

■ IS THE AIRWAY OPEN?

• **Look** for chest and/or abdominal movement, as this will indicate movement of air in and out on inspiration and expiration.

- Consider if the child may have inhaled a foreign body and/or be choking (see Appendix 4 for the Resuscitation Council UK (2010) paediatric FBAO treatment algorithm).

ARE THERE ANY ADDED SOUNDS WHICH MAY INDICATE AIRWAY DIFFICULTIES?

- **Listen** for vocalisations/breath sounds; if present, these will indicate a degree of airway patency, as some air has been able to pass through the vocal cords, generating sound. Common breath sounds include:
  - **stridor** – an abnormal high-pitched sound produced by airflow through a partially obstructed upper airway, often heard in children with croup and indicative of upper airway disease
  - **gurgling** – secretions in the upper airway
  - **snoring** – low-pitched inspiratory sound indicative of partial obstruction in the upper airway, which can be heard in children with large tonsils/adenoids.

Fergusson 2008)
- **Feel** for expired air by placing your cheek over the child's mouth.

AIRWAY ADJUNCTS

Children may require insertion of airway adjuncts to support their airway; these must be inserted by appropriately trained practitioners.

- **Guedel or an oropharyngeal airway.** This may be used in children with a decreased level of consciousness to provide a patent airway. It may not be tolerated by children with a gag reflex. Estimation of size is achieved by placing the flange at the centre of the incisors, with the opposite end reaching the angle of the mandible.

- **Nasopharyngeal airway.** This may be better tolerated than a guedel but is contraindicated in children with basal skull fractures (Advanced Life Support Group 2011). Length is estimated by measuring from the nostrils to the tragus of the ear. A suitable diameter should fit in the nostrils without causing blanching.
- **Endo-tracheal tube.** This provides a passage for gases to flow between a patient's lungs and a breathing system, such as a ventilator circuit or a self-inflating bag valve mask.
- Estimation of the size of uncuffed endo-tracheal tubes for children over 1 is calculated with the following formulas:

Internal diameter (mm) = (Age/4 + 4)
Length (cm) = (Age/2) + 12 – oral tube
Length (cm) = (Age/2 + 15) – nasal tube

(Advanced Life Support Group 2011)

Assessment of Breathing (B)

Primary assessment of the respiratory system involves the following:

- respiratory rate
- recession
- use of accessory muscles
- noises.

Assessment of breathing involves an examination of the **effort**, **efficacy** and **effect** of breathing on other organs (Advanced Life Support Group 2011).

EFFORT OF BREATHING

This is how hard the child is working to achieve their respiratory status.

- Assess respiratory rate, rhythm and depth.
- Respiratory rates are higher in infancy and fall with increasing age as the number and size of alveoli increases with age, providing a greater surface area for gas exchange.
- **Remember: trends rather than absolute values are more valuable, as they provide an indication of improvement or deterioration.**
- **Remember: tachypnoea at rest indicates increased respiratory effort and is usually the first sign of respiratory difficulty.**
- Bradypnoea can indicate fatigue, cerebral depression or a pre-terminal state (Advanced Life Support Group 2011).

Recession

Recession is in-drawing of the muscles of the rib cage, occuring in both infants and children. In older children, this suggests severe respiratory difficulty, as the rib cage is no longer soft and flexible or horizontal, and therefore greater effort is required to cause recession.

- Sites of recession include tracheal tug, suprasternal, clavicular, intercostals, substernal and subcostal (Figure 1).
- Degree of recession indicates severity of respiratory difficulty, as it indicates effort used to draw in muscles.

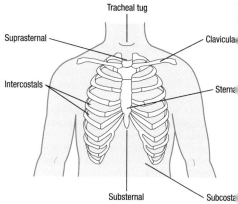

Figure 1 Recession sites

- Sternal recession indicates more severe respiratory distress because the sternum is a large bone and severe effort is being used in order to draw it in.
- Sternal recession and tracheal tug are prominent in upper-airway obstruction (e.g. croup). Lower chest recession indicates lower airway disease (e.g. asthma, bronchiolitis). However, a child in severe respiratory distress may display both upper and lower chest recession, irrespective of the underlying cause.
- **Remember: in an exhausted child, recession decreases.**

Inspiratory and expiratory noises

Noting the characteristics of a noise and when it occurs in the respiratory cycle is an integral part of the respiratory assessment.

- A **wheeze** is a continuous coarse whistling sound which is usually more pronounced on expiration (but can be heard on inspiration), indicating lower-airway narrowing or obstruction. It is common in conditions such as asthma and bronchiolitis.
- **Grunting** is the sound produced when infants close their glottis to keep their alveoli open to prevent airway collapse by creating end expiratory pressure. The same effect is created in older children by breathing with pursed lips.
- **Grunting indicates severe respiratory difficulty → seek immediate medical review.**
- Gasping PRE-TERMINAL WARNING! Gasping is a sign of severe hypoxia and may be pre-terminal.
- **Remember: volume of noise is not an indicator of severity, as it may disappear in the pre-terminal state**.

(Advanced Life Support Group 2011)

Use of accessory muscles

The use of accessory muscles can occur when gas exchange is inadequate due to either increased airway resistance and/or decreased lung compliance (Fergusson 2008).

- Accessory muscles are used to improve the gas exchange.
- Nasal flaring is enlarging of the nostrils on inspiration, which occurs due to reduced airway resistance to maintain airway patency.
- The sternomastoid muscle may be used as an accessory muscle, but in infants it is ineffective and leads to head bobbing with each breath.

- Remember: in the following situations, effort of breathing may not be increased even though the child has breathing difficulty:
  - fatigue/exhaustion
  - reduced respiratory drive, secondary to altered central nervous system (CNS) function
  - neuromuscular disorders.

(Advanced Life Support Group 2011)

In these situations, assessment of efficacy and effect of breathing is important.

■ EFFICACY OF BREATHING

How efficient is the work of breathing? Efficacy of breathing is assessed by inspection and auscultation of the following.

Chest expansion

- This provides an indication that air is being inspired and expired – shallow breathing may lead to hypoxia and ineffective removal of carbon dioxide.
- The degree of chest expansion (or abdominal excursion in infants) should be equal and symmetrical.
- Unequal expansion can indicate pneumothorax, pneumonia, chest trauma, atelectasis and/or inhaled foreign body.

Air entry

- This is assessed by auscultating all lung fields through the entire respiratory cycle.
- Breath sounds should be symmetrical, and present on inspiration and expiration. Decreased breath sounds may indicate obstructed bronchi, hyperinflated lungs, pneumothorax or pleural effusion (Fergusson 2008).

In infants, breath sounds may be louder on auscultation due to their thinner chest wall; sounds are also easily referred because of their small thoracic cavity, leading to difficulties in interpretation (Fergusson 2008).

A **silent chest** may indicate that a child is no longer moving air in and out effectively and is an **extremely worrying sign**. Therefore, **seek emergency help**.

xygen saturation

The normal range is 97–100 per cent in air.

Pulse oximetry provides an estimation of arterial oxygen saturation. **Remember to consider clinical signs and symptoms along with the oxygen saturation reading**.

Always follow manufacturers' and local guidelines when selecting probe size, site and the frequency of site rotation.

Common sites used in young infants are feet, toes and palms, and in older children, fingers and toes.

Remember: a number of factors can impact on the pulse oximeter reading. These include poor perfusion of site area, movement, carbon monoxide poisoning, anaemia and phototherapy.

If pulse oximetry is unavailable, assess the child's nail beds for signs of peripheral cyanosis and look for other signs of poor peripheral perfusion such as cold clammy skin, pallor and mottling. Central cyanosis should be assessed by looking for a bluish tone to the lips.

PRE-TERMINAL WARNING! Central cyanosis is a pre-terminal sign.

Teasdale 2009)

■ EFFECTS OF BREATHING INADEQUACY ON OTHER ORGANS

Heart rate

- Hypoxia can initially lead to a tachycardia, but if it remains uncorrected a bradycardia will occur. **PRE-TERMINAL WARNING!** Bradycardia is a **pre-terminal sign** (Advanced Life Support Group 2011).

Skin colour

- Hypoxia produces vasoconstriction and skin pallor.
- Cyanosis is a late and pre-terminal sign of hypoxia and usually appears only when $SpO_2 \leq 70$ per cent and in the absence of anaemia (Advanced Life Support Group 2011).

Mental status

- Hypoxia can lead to altered mental status: that is, agitation, confusion, drowsiness or altered conscious level.
- These signs of altered mental status in young infants can be difficult to detect. **Remember: parents will often detect subtle changes in their child's mental alertness and condition.**

■ RESPIRATORY SEVERITY ASSESSMENT

Classify the severity of the child's respiratory difficulty in order to trigger and prompt accurate recognition, review and treatment (see Table 4).

Table 4

MODERATE	SEVERE	LIFE THREATENING
• Mild to moderate recession • Babbling/full sentences • O_2 saturations in air 92% or greater	• Severe recession • Short sentences only, too breathless to feed • O_2 saturations < 92% in air • Respiratory rate > 50/min, heart rate > 130 • PFR < 50%	• Severe recession or poor respiratory effort • Too breathless to speak/babble • O_2 saturations < 90% in air • Agitated or drowsy • Exhausted • PFR < 33%

Source / North West and North Wales Critical Care Interface Group (2009). *Guidelines for the Management of Acute Respiratory Failure in Infants and Children.* Reproduced with kind permission.

OXYGEN DELIVERY ADJUNCTS

Children may require oxygen to support oxygenation and ventilation.

Remember: cyanosis that does not correct with oxygen therapy is suggestive of a cardiac abnormality (Advanced Life Support Group 2011). **Seek emergency assessment by medical staff and review the use of oxygen therapy**.

Care needs to be taken to ensure that the right oxygen delivery method is used safely and effectively.

• **Remember: to be effective the method of oxygen delivery is dependent on the oxygen flow rate. If the required flow rate is not set, the oxygen delivery method will not be effective.**

- **Simple face mask:** a plastic mask used to deliver oxygen (O_2) concentrations of between approximately 28 and 50 per cent. Effectiveness of the mask relies on respiratory pattern and a secure fit to prevent leakage. A mask may be poorly tolerated by younger children and limits activities such as communication, eating and drinking. Adhere to manufacturer's guidance regarding flow rates to prevent carbon dioxide retention.

- **Nasal cannula:** a set of two prongs which are placed in the nostrils (ensure the curve of the prong is directed into and naturally lies within the nostrils). The maximum O_2 flow is 2 litres per minute (l.p.m.) in infants and 4 l.p.m. in older children. It allows the child to eat, drink and communicate.

- **Headbox:** a clear perspex box in which only the head and neck of the infant is positioned. Between 21 and 100 per cent oxygen can be administered and must be measured using an oxygen analyser placed near the infant's mouth. Be aware that opening the headbox decreases the oxygen concentration available to the infant. An alternative oxygen delivery method may be needed at this time.

- **Face mask with reservoir bag:** used to deliver high concentrations of oxygen up to 98 per cent, in medical emergencies involving children who are breathing. It requires an oxygen flow rate of between 10 and 15 l.p.m. Oxygen is stored in the reservoir bag during exhalation due to a one-way valve preventing re-breathing of carbon dioxide. The mask should be tight fitting and the reservoir bag should be inflated with oxygen before applying to the child.

- **Bag-valve-mask self-inflating ventilation circuit:** used in medical emergencies involving children who are **not breathing** spontaneously. Attach a face mask that

covers the child's mouth and nose to the circuit.
Manual inflation is required to provide a breath to
the child. Oxygen concentrations of up to 50 per cent
without the reservoir bag and 95 per cent with the
reservoir bag attached can be delivered. **Remember:
it must not be used for 'wafting' oxygen, as there
is a limited oxygen flow if the circuit is not being
manually inflated.**
(Aylott 2010; Fergusson 2008)

Assessment of Circulation (C)

Assessment of circulation involves an examination of
cardiovascular status and the effects of circulatory
inadequacy on other organs.

Primary assessment of the cardiovascular system involves
the following:

• heart rate
• pulse volume
• capillary refill
• blood pressure.

HEART RATE

Heart rate initially increases in the unwell child due to
catecholamine release, which is a compensatory mechanism
for decreased stroke volume. Stroke volume is the amount of
blood that is pumped out by the left ventricle in one contraction.
Infants have a small stroke volume (1.5ml/kg at birth) but the
highest cardiac index (output) during a lifespan (300ml/min/kg).
The cardiac index is reduced to 100ml/min/kg in adolescence
and to 70–80ml/min/kg in the adult. As the heart gets larger,

stroke volume increases. Cardiac output is the result of stroke volume and heart rate, which are represented in the heart rate differences of childhood.

- The heart rate in infants can be extremely high (up to 220 beats per minute). A consistently high heart rate can lead to exhaustion and bradycardia.
- PRE-TERMINAL WARNING! **Bradycardia and exhaustion are pre-terminal signs.**

■ PULSE VOLUME

Pulse volume/matter (or strength) gives an indication of heart function and cardiac output. The strength of the pulse is determined by the force of the left ventricle contraction and the stroke volume.

- Pulse volume is assessed by palpating and comparing both peripheral (radial) and central pulses (carotid/brachial/femoral).
- A bounding pulse may be a result of increased cardiac output (as in septicaemia), hypercapnia or arteriovenous systemic shunt.
- A weak, thready pulse can indicate cold shock, hypotension and/or heart failure.
- PRE-TERMINAL WARNING! **Absent peripheral and weak central pulses are signs of advanced shock and are a pre-terminal sign.**

■ PULSE RHYTHM

A normal heart rate heard on auscultation is a regular 'lub-dub' where two heart sounds are heard (S_I and S_{II}). These are generated by the normal heart valves closing while the heart pumps.

- Hearing the third heart sound (S_{III}) in children can be normal, but a fourth heart sound (S_{IV}) is abnormal. This sound is rarely heard but could indicate heart failure and is referred to as 'gallop rhythm'.
- Gallop rhythm can be difficult to detect when the child has a high heart rate. If detected, additional signs and symptoms of heart failure need to be considered such as poor feeding (infants), lethargy, sweating, shortness of breath, cold and clammy peripheries, and pallor.
- A heart murmur is an additional sound heard in between the 'lub-dub', characterised by an accentuated and elongated 'swishing' sound.
- Most murmurs are innocent and may be detected during a routine examination and come and go during childhood.
- An innocent murmur may be accentuated if the child has a fever or is tachycardic.
- A murmur can be indicative of a congenital heart defect and additional investigations may need to be performed (e.g. echocardiogram).

CAPILLARY REFILL TIME (CRT) AND BODY TEMPERATURE

CRT should be assessed by two methods:

- Central – press with one finger in the centre of the sternum for 5 seconds and release.
- Peripheral – elevate a digit to above heart level, press on the digit for 5 seconds and release.
- CRT should be < 2 seconds. An increase in CRT indicates poor perfusion and can be an early sign of septic shock.
- **PRE-TERMINAL WARNING!** Central cyanosis is a pre-terminal sign and cardiorespiratory arrest is imminent.

- **Remember: the ambient temperature must be considered when assessing capillary refill time, particularly following trauma where the child has been exposed to a cold environment.**
- Additional signs of poor perfusion are cold and clammy skin, pallor, mottling and peripheral cyanosis.

■ BLOOD PRESSURE

A blood pressure reading should always be taken as a baseline. Initially this will be a non-invasive measurement, using a sphygmomanometer or an oscillometric device (e.g. Dinamap). Invasive arterial blood pressure monitoring is performed in those children who are critically unwell and require an arterial line for arterial blood gas sampling.

- When cardiac output is decreased, children and infants initiate compensatory mechanisms (vasoconstriction, tachycardia and increased cardiac contractility) which help to maintain blood pressure. **Remember: once the compensatory mechanisms begin to fail, the blood pressure starts to decrease.**
- PRE-TERMINAL WARNING! Hypotension is often a late sign of circulatory failure in the child.

■ RECOGNISING THE SHOCKED CHILD

Shock is a life-threatening condition with a variety of causes. It is characterised by an inability of the circulatory system to supply adequate oxygen and nutrients to the tissues, and to excrete waste products.

To supply adequate nutrition to the tissues, the following are needed:

- cardiac pump (heart)

- circulatory system with no obstruction to the flow
- adequate blood volume.

If any of the above is impaired, a cascade of responses is triggered:

cellular starvation → cell death → organ dysfunction → organ failure → death

(Advanced Life Support Group, 2011)

■ CLASSIFICATION AND CAUSES OF SHOCK

The most common examples of presenting conditions are emboldened in Table 5.

Table 5

CLASSIFICATION	CAUSE	EXAMPLES
Hypovolaemic	Loss of fluid	**Haemorrhage**, **gastroenteritis**, **intussuseption**, burns, peritonitis
Distributive	Vascular failure	**Septicaemia**, anaphylaxis
Cardiogenic	Pump failure	Arrhythmia, heart failure, cardiomyopathy
Obstructive	Flow restriction	Tension pneumothorax, haemo-pneumothorax, flail chest, congenital cardiac disease
Dissociative	Red cell failure	Profound anaemia, carbon monoxide poisoning

Reference / Advanced Life Support Group (2011).

■ THE THREE STAGES OF SHOCK (see Table 6)

1 Compensated shock (early stage)

- The causative mechanism of shock triggers a number of compensatory mechanisms in order to maintain perfusion of the vital organs (heart, brain and kidneys).
- The main hormone involved in this response is adrenaline but other hormones such as noradrenaline, cortisol and adrenocorticotrophic hormone (ACTH) are also activated.
- This process is commonly referred to as 'fight or flight'.

2 Uncompensated shock

- If early-stage shock is not treated then the compensatory mechanisms identified above begin to fail and the severity of shock progresses further.

3 Irreversible shock

- If shock goes untreated it will progress to this phase and death is inevitable.
- The diagnosis is a retrospective one.
- The cellular damage cannot be reversed and multiple organ failure has occurred.
- **Remember: shock is a progressive condition and early recognition is vital to prevent progression from compensated to uncompensated shock.**

Table 6

INCREASING SEVERITY OF PHYSIOLOGICAL SHOCK		

COMPENSATED	UNCOMPENSATED	IRREVERSIBLE
• Normal BP • Tachycardia • Increased, shallow respiratory rate due to ↑ metabolic acidosis • ↑ CRT Cold/clammy peripheries (blood vessels supplying non-vital organs constrict; skin and blood volume conserved for vital organs, e.g. heart and brain) • Possible agitation, anxiety or confusion due to mild hypoxia • Urine output decreased (< 1ml/kg in children and < 2ml/kg in infants) • Increase in enzymes (angiotension and vasopressin) forces kidneys to conserve water and salt	• Falling BP **PRE-TERMINAL WARNING!** • Tachycardia • Acidotic breathing (deep, laboured and gasping) – to exhale excess CO_2 • CRT time remains prolonged despite fluid boluses • Depressed cerebral state • Reduced/absent urine output	• Hypotensive • Bradycardia • Respiratory/cardiac arrest • Multiple organ failure • Diagnosis is retrospective • Death inevitable

Reference / Advanced Life Support Group (2011).

■ MENINGOCOCCAL SEPTICAEMIA: SIGNS AND SYMPTOMS

Meningococcal infection is caused by the *Neisseria meningitidis* bacterium. It is a life-threatening disease that causes inflammation of the meninges (lining of the brain) and septicaemia (blood poisoning). **Early recognition is vital.**

- The key sign of meningococcal septicaemia is the presence of a purpuric rash in the unwell child.
- A blanching pink rash that fades under pressure is present initially in up to 30 per cent of cases, which then develops into a purpuric rash (Meningitis Research Foundation, 2009)
- Alert or red flag symptoms of septicaemia and circulatory shut down are: pale or mottled skin, limb pain and cold extremities. These signs can appear 5 hours or more earlier than the classic symptoms (rash, neck stiffness and photophobia) (Meningitis Research Foundation, 2009).
- Signs and symptoms of meningococcal septicaemia are:
  - Clinically shocked
  - Rash – this may vary and may not even be present initially. It will range from pinprick petechiae or a viral blanching rash to large purpuric spots. In only 7 per cent of cases a rash does **not** appear (Advanced Life Support Group, 2011)
  - Fever
  - Muscle aches and pains
  - Lethargy
  - Abdominal pain, diarrhoea and vomiting
  - Altered mental state
  - Respiratory signs and symptoms
  - Appears unwell
  - Refusing to eat/drink.
  (Advanced Life Support Group 2011; NICE 2010)

RECOGNISING THE DEHYDRATED CHILD

NICE (2009) has produced guidelines on the recognition of worsening dehydration for children under 5 with diarrhoea and vomiting (see Table 7).

Additional clinical signs of dehydration are:

- weight loss (although a pre-sickness weight is not often available)
- sunken fontanelle (in children < 18–24 months old)

(Advanced Life Support Group, 2011)

Table 7

Symptoms (remote and face-to-face assessment)	INCREASING SEVERITY OF SHOCK →		
	No clinically detectable dehydration	Clinical dehydration	Clinical shock
	Appears well	Appears to be unwell or deteriorating ⚐	–
	Alert and responsive	Altered responsiveness (e.g. irritable, lethargic) ⚐	Decreased level of consciousness
	Normal urine output	Decreased urine output	–
	Skin colour unchanged	Skin colour unchanged	Pale or mottled skin
	Warm extremities	Warm extremities	Cold extremities

⇒

INCREASING SEVERITY OF SHOCK		

Signs (face-to-face assessment)	Alert and responsive	Altered responsiveness (e.g. irritable, lethargic) 🏳	Decreased level of consciousness
	Skin colour unchanged	Skin colour unchanged	Pale or mottled skin
	Warm extremities	Warm extremities	Cold extremities
	Eyes not sunken	Sunken eyes 🏳	–
	Moist mucous membranes (except after a drink)	Dry mucous membranes (except for 'mouth breathers')	–
	Normal heart rate	Tachycardia 🏳	Tachycardia
	Normal breathing pattern	Tachypnoea 🏳	Tachypnoea
	Normal peripheral pulses	Normal peripheral pulses	Weak peripheral pulses
	Normal capillary refill time	Normal capillary refill time	Prolonged capillary refill time
	Normal skin turgor	Reduced skin turgor 🏳	–
	Normal blood pressure	Normal blood pressure	Hypotension (decompensated shock)

Note: The flag (🏳) represents those children who are potentially at risk of progression to clinical shock.

Source / National Institute for Health and Clinical Excellence (2009). *CG 84 Diarrhoea and Vomiting in Children under 5.* London: NICE. Available from: www.nice.org.uk/guidance/CG84. Reproduced with kind permission.

CALCULATION OF FLUID REQUIREMENTS

- The child with dehydration and no shock is assumed to be 5 per cent dehydrated.
- If the child is clinically shocked then 10 per cent dehydration or greater has occurred.
- Management of dehydration consists of an initial fluid bolus (20 ml/kg). This is followed by the administration of the calculated daily maintenance fluids **added to** the calculated replacement fluids delivered over 24 hours (Table 8).

(Advanced Life Support Group 2011)

Table 8

BODY WEIGHT	FLUID REQUIREMENT PER DAY (ML/KG)	FLUID REQUIREMENT PER HOUR (ML/KG)
First 10 kg	100	4
Second 10 kg	50	2
Subsequent kgs	20	1

Source / Advanced Life Support Group, *Advanced Paediatric Life Support: The Practical Approach*, 5th Edition. Copyright © 2011 by Wiley-Blackwell. Reprinted by permission of John Wiley & Sons, Inc.

Replacement fluids are calculated by the following formula:
- 100 ml/kg for 10 per cent dehydrated
- 50 ml/kg for 5 per cent dehydrated

(Advanced Life Support Group, 2011)

Example

A 12 kg child is estimated to be 10 per cent dehydrated from their signs and symptoms.
Fluid bolus: 20 ml/kg = $20 \times 12 = $ **240 ml**
Fluid therapy over 24 hours = Replacement + Maintenance
Replacement $100 \times 12 = 1200$ ml added to:
Maintenance 1100 ml = **2300 ml in 24 hours**

Assessment of Disability (D)

■ RAPID ASSESSMENT OF DISABILITY: AVPU

Remember: neurological conditions may impact on respiration and circulation, and in turn respiratory and circulatory problems may manifest in neurological symptoms. Assessment of disability (D) should therefore be conducted only after assessing and securing management of the airway (A), breathing (B) and circulation (C).

- A rapid initial assessment of the child's conscious level can be assessed using the AVPU scale.

A = **Alert**
V = responds to **Voice**
P = responds to **Pain**
U = **Unresponsive** to all stimuli

- If the child is not alert, a vocal prompt should be given, such as calling the child's name. If the child does not respond to voice then a painful stimulus should be applied, recording limb, eye and vocal reactions, as these will indicate the severity of the child's condition and the equivalent Glasgow Coma Scale (GCS) score (Advanced Life Support Group 2011).
- **A child who is not assessed as alert using the AVPU scale should be considered to have some degree of neurological compromise.**
- A child who is not alert but responds to voice is considered to have an equivalent GCS of 11 → **seek immediate medical review** (Cockett and Day 2010).

If the child is unresponsive to voice, a central painful stimulus must be applied in the form of either a sternal rub or pulling frontal hair. Supraorbital ridge pressure may also be applied as a central painful stimulus **but** should only be performed by those specifically trained and competent to do so (Advanced Life Support Group 2011).

Upon application of a painful stimulus, a child should localise to pain: reach for and purposefully locate the site of the pain and try to remove the painful source. An infant cannot localise to pain and instead should withdraw from the painful stimulus.

The child may also demonstrate localising to the point of pain by purposefully reaching out, locating and pulling at equipment, probes and intravenous lines which may be a source of irritation to them. Record and report all such activity (Cockett and Day 2010).

Remember: a peripheral stimulus may only elicit a spinal reflex, which may not reflect the child's brain function accurately. A central painful stimulus is therefore regarded as a more accurate method of eliciting a response from a child in a deep coma (Warren 2010).

Application of a painful stimulus may cause bruising and appear to cause distress to the child. Prior to applying the stimulus, prepare the parents by explaining the importance and purpose of the procedure. Record the site of the stimulus and rotate sites in an attempt to prevent bruising.

- A child who is responsive to pain only is considered to have an equivalent GCS of 8 or below and is therefore at high risk of airway compromise → **best practice guidance indicates that emergency intubation and ventilation is required** (NICE 2007b).
- The unresponsive but breathing child is considered to have an equivalent GCS of 3 with cardiorespiratory arrest imminent → **ensure a cardiac arrest call is made and resuscitation is commenced** (Cockett and Day 2010).

■ POSTURE

Assessment of posture (either immediately observable or elicited by a painful stimulus) can provide a quickly recognisable indication of the severity of the child's condition:

- **Hypotonic posture:** children with serious illness very often present with a 'floppy' and lifeless posture; they act out of character by offering little or no objection to painful procedures, lying quietly and appearing exhausted. PRE-TERMINAL WARNING! Exhaustion is a pre-terminal sign – collapse is imminent → seek emergency help.
- **Opisthotonos:** the back arches and the neck is extended due to meningeal irritation: it is a worrying sign → **seek urgent medical review.** Take care not to mistake opisthotonos for hyperextension of the neck due to upper-airway obstruction.
- **Abnormal flexion/decorticate posture:** a stiff posture demonstrating arms flexed towards the chest; wrists may rotate inwards towards the chest and thumbs may flex over the fingers; the legs remain extended. This is a sign of raised intracranial pressure and may indicate a poor outcome.

Abnormal extension/decerebrate posture: a stiff posture demonstrating extended arms and legs; shoulders may rotate inwards with hands rotating outwards. This is a sign of raised intracranial pressure and may indicate a poor outcome.

Take care not to mistake decorticate or decerebrate postures for the tonic phase of a convulsion.

(Advanced Life Support Group 2011)

PUPILS

Pupil reactions indicate oculomotor nerve function and intracranial pressure (ICP). Pupils should be equal in size and react briskly to light.

Most concerning pupillary signs are dilatation, inequality and sluggish or unreactive pupils, as they are suggestive of raised intracranial pressure → seek emergency help.

Fixed dilated pupils: a very worrying sign which may be indicative of brainstem herniation (coning), leading to death. Fixed dilated pupils may also be observed during and after seizures, as a result of hypothermia or as the side-effect of some drugs.

Pinpoint pupils: may indicate ingestion of opiates or metabolic dysfunction.

Unequal pupil size or reaction: the side of the abnormal pupil reaction indicates the side of the brain affected (e.g. left pupil inequality indicates a problem in the left side of the brain). Some children may have a misshaped pupil – check with parents to avoid misinterpretation of normal features.

(Advanced Life Support Group 2011; Warren 2010)

■ CAUSES OF RAISED INTRACRANIAL PRESSURE

Intracranial pressure (ICP) is the pressure within the skull. The skull is a rigid structure containing three components: the brain, cerebrospinal fluid and blood. An increase in volume in any of these component parts without a compensatory decrease in another will lead to raised intracranial pressure, causing a reduction in cerebral blood flow and perfusion. There is little room within the skull following closure of the fontanelles to accommodate any sustained extra volume (Waterhouse 2005).

Causes of raised intracranial pressure include:

- **Space-occupying lesions:** such as a tumour, haematom or abscess.
- **Cerebral oedema:** can occur as a result of metabolic factors, hypercapnia (raised carbon dioxide in the blood, causing vasodilation of cerebral vessels) and head injury.
- **An increase in CSF production:** can occur in meningitis and subarachnoid haemorrhage.
- **Obstruction to CSF flow and absorption:** increases the volume of CSF, as can occur in hydrocephalus.
- **Obstructed venous return** causing intracranial pressure to rise: can occur due to an embolism or thrombus.

(Cockett and Day 2010; Waterhouse 2005)

■ SIGNS OF RAISED INTRACRANIAL PRESSURE

Specifically observe for signs of raised intracranial pressure as part of the assessment of disability (Table 9).

Table 9

EARLY SIGNS OF RAISED INTRACRANIAL PRESSURE	LATE SIGNS OF RAISED INTRACRANIAL PRESSURE

• Drowsiness → reduced level of consciousness (LOC)
• Irritability
• Headache
• High-pitched cry (infants)
• Bulging fontanelle (infants)
• Papilloedema
• Nausea and vomiting
• Seizures
• Abnormal pupil responses:
  – dilatation
  – sluggish reaction
  – inequality in size and reaction
	• Pupil(s) becoming increasingly large with decreased response to light (known as a 'blown' pupil)
	• Fixed dilated pupils – which may be indicative of brain-stem herniation 'coning', leading to death
	• Abnormal posture which may be immediately observable or elicited by a painful stimulus:
	  – decorticate (abnormal flexion)
	  – decerebrate (abnormal extension)
	• **Cushing's triad = bradycardia, hypertension and respiratory depression** `PRE-TERMINAL WARNING!` → a very late sign indicating severe and irreversible brain damage with a high risk of mortality

References / Advanced Life Support Group (2011); Cockett and Day (2010); Dixon and Murphy (2009); Fergusson (2008).

■ SEIZURES

Many seizures in children have no identifiable cause. However, some causes include: febrile convulsions; toxicity (poisons/alcohol/drugs); head/brain trauma; metabolic disorders (hypoglycaemia/electrolyte imbalance); brain lesions (tumours/bleeds/abscesses); infection/sepsis.

Observe for signs of seizure activity such as:

- limb rigidity and muscle contraction (as seen during the tonic phase of a seizure)
- jerking of muscles (as seen during the clonic phase of a seizure)
- auras/vacancy
- twitching or spasms
- transient weakness and/or dysphasia that may be observable post-seizure
- spontaneous startle-like movements.

Remember that signs of seizure activity may be subtle, especially in infants due to the immaturity of the brain, **making it easy to miss them** (Dixon and Murphy 2009).

■ 'DON'T EVER FORGET GLUCOSE': DEFG

Check blood glucose as a matter of routine, using both a glucose test stick and laboratory analysis.

- Treatment for hypoglycaemia (blood glucose < 3 mmol/l): intravenous bolus dose 2 ml/kg of 10 per cent glucose followed by an infusion containing glucose.

(Advanced Life Support Group 2011)

◀ TIPS TO PROMOTE ACCURATE MEASUREMENT AND RECORDING OF NEUROLOGICAL OBSERVATIONS

Neurological observations are a sensitive indicator of neurological functioning and deterioration, aiding early recognition of the acutely ill child. Assessment and interpretation of neurological function in children is complex, warranting precision and accuracy in the measurement and recording of neurological observations. Do not undertake neurological observations unless specifically trained and competent to do so: seek immediate help if unsure.

Use an age-appropriate coma scale specifically adapted for use with children.

A good understanding of normal child development is required in order to distinguish abnormal responses.

Check whether the child is on any medication or has a pre-existing condition or any developmental delay that may impact on normal ranges. These need to be considered when interpreting observations.

Perform your first set of neurological observations with the previous assessor to check and confirm interpretation of the observations made.

Consider the impact that unfamiliar surroundings and fear may have on the child's behaviour and level of co-operation.

The sleeping child needs to be roused prior to neurological assessment.

Record the size and equality of the pupils **prior to** shining a light in the eyes.

- As well as checking for individual pupil response to light, check consensual response – shining the light into one pupil should also make the other pupil constrict.
- Document which painful stimulus is used, to aid consistency, protect sites and improve interpretation.
- Involve other more senior colleagues in the interpretation of the observations.

(Dixon and Murphy 2009; Fergusson 2008; Warren 2010)

■ CONTRAINDICATIONS TO PERFORMING A LUMBAR PUNCTURE

For diagnostic purposes it may be necessary to perform a lumbar puncture. There is a risk of brainstem death (coning), leading to death, if a lumbar puncture is performed on a child with signs of raised intracranial pressure. Assessment of the child prior to the procedure is therefore vital. A lumbar puncture should **not** be performed in the following circumstances:

- if signs of raised intracranial pressure are present
- if coma is observed
- if the GCS score is 13 or less
- if the child has a coagulation disorder
- if any signs of seizure are present
- if there is respiratory depression
- in the acutely ill child if there is a purpuric rash/signs of meningococcal disease, dehydration or shock
- when there is a suspicion of or confirmed C spine injury (due to the position required by the procedure).

(Advanced Life Support Group 2011; Pettit 2010)

ssessment of Exposure (E)

ook for signs of a rash, isolated spots or bruises, however
mall, because they may be significant to the early diagnosis
f specific conditions or identification of safeguarding issues.
arly diagnosis and treatment are essential to improving
atient outcomes. Record all blemishes, bruises and rashes
n a body chart.

RASHES AND BRUISING

Petechiae (purple/pink pinprick spots which become
non-blanching) and purpura (red/purple blemishes or
bruising under the skin which become non-blanching)
are indicative of septicaemia.

Urticaria (raised red blotches) are indicative of an allergic
reaction.

Maculopapular rash (small flat red spots with raised
bumps) are indicative of an allergic reaction, measles
or sepsis.

dvanced Life Support Group 2011)

TEMPERATURE

A fever may indicate an infection.

Prolonged seizures or shivering may also give rise to a
fever (Advanced Life Support Group 2011).

Listen to parents – measure the child's temperature when
parents express concern; they may notice subtle signs
that the child's temperature is increasing before planned
measurement is due to take place.

Appendix 1: Physiological observations: normal ranges and estimation of weight formula

■ NORMAL RANGES

AGE (YEARS)	HEART RATE	RESPIRATORY RATE	SYSTOLIC BP (mmHg) 5TH CENTILE	SYSTOLIC BP (mmHg) 50TH CENTILE
< 1	110–160	30–40	65–75	80–90
1–2	100–150	25–35	70–75	85–95
2–5	95–140	25–30	70–80	85–100
5–12	80–120	20–25	80–90	90–110
> 12	60–100	15–20	90–105	100–120

Source / Advanced Life Support Group, *Advanced Paediatric Life Support: The Practical Approach*, 5th Edition. Copyright © 2011 by Wiley-Blackwell. Reprinted by permission of John Wiley & Sons, Inc.

■ ESTIMATION OF WEIGHT FORMULA

WORKS BEST FOR	FORMULA
0–12 months	Weight (kg) = (0.5 × age in months) + 4
1–5 years	Weight (kg) = (2 × age in years) + 8
6–12 years	Weight (kg) = (3 × age in years) + 7

Reference / Advanced Life Support Group (2011).

ppendix 2: Paediatric SBAR tool

S

Situation:
I am (name), a nurse on ward (X)
I am calling about (child X)
I am calling because I am concerned that . . .
(e.g. BP is low/high, pulse is XXX temperature is XX,
Early Warning Score is XX)

B

Background:
Child (X) was admitted on (XX date) with
(e.g. respiratory infection)
They have had (X operation/procedure/investigation)
Child (X)'s condition has changed in the last (XX mins)
Their last set of obs were (XXX)
The child's normal condition is . . .
(e.g. alert/drowsy/confused, pain free)

A

Assessment:
I think the problem is (XXX)
and I have . . .
(e.g. given O_2/analgesia, stopped the infusion)
OR
I am not sure what the problem is but child (X) is deteriorating
OR
I don't know what's wrong but I am really worried

R

Recommendation:
I need you to . . .
Come to see the child in the next (XX mins)
AND
Is there anything I need to do in the meantime?
(e.g. stop the fluid/repeat the obs)

Ask receiver to repeat key information to ensure understanding

ource / The Paediatric SBAR card design is reproduced by permission of the NHS Institute for
nnovation and Improvement, Coventry, England, www.institute.nhs.uk. The SBAR tool originated
om the US Navy and was adapted for use in healthcare by Dr M. Leonard and colleagues from
aiser Permanente, Colorado, USA.

Appendix 3: Basic life support – paediatric algorithm

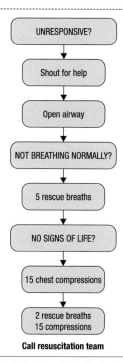

UNRESPONSIVE?

↓

Shout for help

↓

Open airway

↓

NOT BREATHING NORMALLY?

↓

5 rescue breaths

↓

NO SIGNS OF LIFE?

↓

15 chest compressions

↓

2 rescue breaths
15 compressions

Call resuscitation team

Source / Reproduced with the kind permission of the Resuscitation Council (UK).

ppendix 4: Paediatric FBAO treatment algorithm

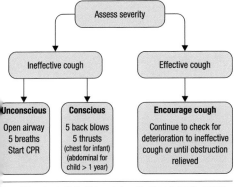

Assess severity

Ineffective cough | Effective cough

Unconscious
Open airway
5 breaths
Start CPR

Conscious
5 back blows
5 thrusts
(chest for infant)
(abdominal for
child > 1 year)

Encourage cough
Continue to check for
deterioration to ineffective
cough or until obstruction
relieved

ource / Reproduced with the kind permission of the Resuscitation Council (UK).

eferences

dvanced Life Support Group (2011) *Advanced Paediatric
Life Support: The Practical Approach*, 5th edn. Chichester:
Wiley-Blackwell.

ylott, M. (2010) Non-invasive respiratory therapy. In
Glasper, A.; Aylott, M. and Battrick, C. (eds), *Developing
Practical Skills for Nursing Children and Young People*.
London: Hodder Arnold, pp. 357–70.

EMACH (2008) *Why Children Die: A Pilot Study 2006,
Children and Young People's Report*. London:
Confidential Enquiry into Maternal and Child Health.

Cockett, A. and Day, H. (eds) (2010) *Children's High Dependency Nursing.* Chichester: Wiley-Blackwell.

Dixon, M. and Murphy, J. (2009) The child with acute neurological dysfunction. In Dixon, M.; Crawford, D.; Teasdale, D. and Murphy, J. (eds), *Nursing the Highly Dependent Child or Infant: A Manual of Care.* Chichester: Wiley-Blackwell, pp. 129–50.

Dougherty, L. and Lister, S. (eds) (2008) *The Royal Marsden Manual of Clinical Nursing Procedures: Student Edition.* Chichester: Wiley-Blackwell.

Fergusson, D. (2008) *Clinical Assessment and Monitoring in Children.* Oxford: Blackwell.

Glasper, A.; McEwing, G. and Richardson, J. (2007) *Oxford Handbook of Children's and Young People's Nursing.* Oxford: Oxford University Press.

Glasper, A.; McEwing, G. and Richardson, J. (2011) *Emergencies in Children's and Young People's Nursing.* Oxford: Oxford University Press.

Meningitis Research Foundation (2009) *Early Recognition of Meningitis and Septicaemia.* Bristol: Meningitis Research Foundation.

NICE (2007a) *Feverish illness in children: Assessment and initial management in children younger than 5 years. NICE Clinical Guideline 47.* London: National Institute for Health and Clinical Excellence.

NICE (2007b) *Head injury: Triage, assessment, investigation and early management of head injury in infants, children and adults. NICE Clinical Guideline 56.* London: National Institute for Health and Clinical Excellence.

CE (2009) *Diarrhoea and vomiting in children under 5. NICE Clinical Guideline 84.* London: National Institute for Health and Clinical Excellence.

CE (2010) *Bacterial meningitis and meningococcal septicaemia: Management of bacterial meningitis and meningococcal septicaemia in children and young people younger than 16 years in primary and secondary care. NICE Clinical Guideline 102.* London: National Institute for Health and Clinical Excellence.

PSA (2007) *Recognising and responding appropriately to early signs of deterioration in hospitalised patients.* London: National Patient Safety Agency.

ettit, G. (2010) Lumbar puncture. In Trigg, E. and Mohammed, T. A. (eds), *Practices in Children's Nursing: Guidelines for Hospital and Community*, 3rd edn. London: Churchill Livingstone/Elsevier, pp. 175–81.

CN (2011) *Standards for assessing, measuring and monitoring vital signs in infants, children and young people.* London: Royal College of Nursing.

easdale, D. (2009) Physiological monitoring. In Dixon, M.; Crawford, D.; Teasdale, D. and Murphy, J. (eds), *Nursing the Highly Dependent Child or Infant: A Manual of Care.* Chichester: Wiley-Blackwell, pp. 13–45.

he Resuscitation Council (UK) (2010) *Paediatric Basic Life Support (Healthcare Professionals with a Duty to Respond) Algorithm.* London: Resuscitation Council (UK).

he Resuscitation Council (UK) (2010) *Paediatric FBAO Treatment Algorithm.* London: Resuscitation Council (UK).

Warren, A. (2010) Neurological observations and coma scale In Trigg, E. and Mohammed, T. A. (eds), *Practices in Children Nursing: Guidelines for Hospital and Community*, 3rd edn London: Churchill Livingstone/Elsevier, pp. 182–94.

Waterhouse, C. (2005) The Glasgow Coma Scale and other neurological observations. *Nursing Standard*, vol. 19, no. 33, pp. 56–64.

Useful websites

Advanced Life Support Group (ALSG):
www.alsg.org/en

British Thoracic Society:
www.brit-thoracic.org.uk

European Resuscitation Council (ERC):
www.erc.edu/index.php/mainpage/en

Meningitis Research Foundation:
www.meningitis.org

Meningitis UK:
www.meningitisuk.org

National Institute for Health and Clinical Excellence:
www.nice.org.uk

National Patient Safety Agency:
www.npsa.nhs.uk

Resuscitation Council (UK):
www.resus.org.uk/SiteIndx.htm

Spotting the Sick Child:
www.spottingthesickchild.com